Consultations & Appointments

Form Organiser

for Indian Head Massage Therapists

by Galina St George

Therapist name......................................

Address..

....

Telephone number...................................

Appointments

Name	Phone Number	Date/ Time	Notes

Appointments

Name	Phone Number	Date/ Time	Notes

Appointments

Name	Phone Number	Date/ Time	Notes

Appointments

Name	Phone Number	Date/Time	Notes

Appointments

Name	Phone Number	Date/ Time	Notes

Appointments

Name	Phone Number	Date/ Time	Notes

Appointments

Name	Phone Number	Date/Time	Notes

INDIAN HEAD MASSAGE CONSULTATION FORM

Therapist:	Therapist's address:	Date:
Client's name	Age	Gender
Client's address:

Tel No: | Occupation: | Doctor's address/Telephone No. : |

CONTRA-INDICATIONS

Diabetes	Cuts / Abrasions/recent scars	Spastic conditions
Abnormal blood pressure	Migraine	Sties
Epilepsy	Osteoporosis	Conjunctivitis
Cancer	Local infections	Advanced asthma
Undiagnosed lumps	Contagious skin disorders	Herpes Simplex
Thrombosis / Embolism	Fractures / Sprains	Other

CAUTIONS

Thrombosis/Strokes	Osteoporosis	Back/Neck problems
Aneurosa	Spondilitis	Recent operations
M.E.	Thyroid problems	Medication taken

LIFESTYLE / OTHER DETAILS

Occupation		Sleep patterns	
General Health		Allergies	
Exercise		Medication taken	
Diet		History of headaches/ migraines	
Fluid intake (water,		Emotional /	

juice)		psychological state at present	
Smoking		Stress levels	
Alcohol		Methods of relaxation	

OBJECTIVES OF THE TREATMENT & TREATMENT PLAN

What does the client hope to achieve?	
What will it be possible to achieve realistically? (Short term and long-term goals)	
Treatment plan agreed with the client (number of treatments to be given, over what period of time, length of time between treatments, areas to be paid particular attention to during the treatments)	

DISCLAIMER

I declare, that all the information regarding me in this form is true and accurate, and as far as I am aware, I can undertake a massage treatment without any adverse effects. I have been fully informed of any contra-indications and I am willing to undertake the treatment with this therapist.

Client's signature..Date...

TREATMENT DETAILS & CLIENT RESPONSE TO TREATMENT

Medium used:

Treatment 1 / Date...

Treatment 2 / Date...

Treatment 3 / Date...

Treatment 4 / Date...

Client's response / reactions to the treatments:

Treatment 1 / Date..

Treatment 2 / Date..

Treatment 3 / Date..

Treatment 4 / Date..

AFTERCARE AND GENERAL ADVICE

Treatment 1..

Treatment 2 ....

Treatment 3 ....

Treatment 4 ....

CLIENT'S FEEDBACK/ COMMENTS

Signature .... Date..

INDIAN HEAD MASSAGE CONSULTATION FORM

Therapist:	Therapist's address:	Date:
Client's name	Age	Gender
Client's address: Tel No:	Occupation:	Doctor's address/Telephone No. :

CONTRA-INDICATIONS

Diabetes	Cuts / Abrasions/recent scars	Spastic conditions
Abnormal blood pressure	Migraine	Sties
Epilepsy	Osteoporosis	Conjunctivitis
Cancer	Local infections	Advanced asthma
Undiagnosed lumps	Contagious skin disorders	Herpes Simplex
Thrombosis / Embolism	Fractures / Sprains	Other

CAUTIONS

Thrombosis/Strokes	Osteoporosis	Back/Neck problems
Aneurosa	Spondilitis	Recent operations
M.E.	Thyroid problems	Medication taken

LIFESTYLE / OTHER DETAILS

Occupation		Sleep patterns	
General Health		Allergies	
Exercise		Medication taken	
Diet		History of headaches/ migraines	
Fluid intake (water,		Emotional /	

juice)		psychological state at present	
Smoking		Stress levels	
Alcohol		Methods of relaxation	

OBJECTIVES OF THE TREATMENT & TREATMENT PLAN

What does the client hope to achieve?	
What will it be possible to achieve realistically? (Short term and long-term goals)	
Treatment plan agreed with the client (number of treatments to be given, over what period of time, length of time between treatments, areas to be paid particular attention to during the treatments)	

DISCLAIMER

I declare, that all the information regarding me in this form is true and accurate, and as far as I am aware, I can undertake a massage treatment without any adverse effects. I have been fully informed of any contra-indications and I am willing to undertake the treatment with this therapist.

Client's signature...Date...

TREATMENT DETAILS & CLIENT RESPONSE TO TREATMENT

Medium used:

Treatment 1 / Date...

Treatment 2 / Date...

Treatment 3 / Date...

Treatment 4 / Date...

Client's response / reactions to the treatments:

Treatment 1 / Date...

Treatment 2 / Date...

Treatment 3 / Date...

Treatment 4 / Date...

AFTERCARE AND GENERAL ADVICE

Treatment 1..

Treatment 2..

Treatment 3..

Treatment 4..

CLIENT'S FEEDBACK/ COMMENTS

Signature .... Date...

INDIAN HEAD MASSAGE CONSULTATION FORM

Therapist:	Therapist's address:	Date:
Client's name	Age	Gender
Client's address: Tel No:	Occupation:	Doctor's address/Telephone No. :

CONTRA-INDICATIONS

Diabetes	Cuts / Abrasions/recent scars	Spastic conditions
Abnormal blood pressure	Migraine	Sties
Epilepsy	Osteoporosis	Conjunctivitis
Cancer	Local infections	Advanced asthma
Undiagnosed lumps	Contagious skin disorders	Herpes Simplex
Thrombosis / Embolism	Fractures / Sprains	Other

CAUTIONS

Thrombosis/Strokes	Osteoporosis	Back/Neck problems
Aneurosa	Spondilitis	Recent operations
M.E.	Thyroid problems	Medication taken

LIFESTYLE / OTHER DETAILS

Occupation		Sleep patterns	
General Health		Allergies	
Exercise		Medication taken	
Diet		History of headaches/ migraines	
Fluid intake (water,		Emotional /	

juice)		psychological state at present	
Smoking		Stress levels	
Alcohol		Methods of relaxation	

OBJECTIVES OF THE TREATMENT & TREATMENT PLAN

What does the client hope to achieve?	
What will it be possible to achieve realistically? (Short term and long-term goals)	
Treatment plan agreed with the client (number of treatments to be given, over what period of time, length of time between treatments, areas to be paid particular attention to during the treatments)	

DISCLAIMER

I declare, that all the information regarding me in this form is true and accurate, and as far as I am aware, I can undertake a massage treatment without any adverse effects. I have been fully informed of any contra-indications and I am willing to undertake the treatment with this therapist.

Client's signature..Date...

TREATMENT DETAILS & CLIENT RESPONSE TO TREATMENT

Medium used:

Treatment 1 / Date..

Treatment 2 / Date..

Treatment 3 / Date..

Treatment 4 / Date..

Client's response / reactions to the treatments:

Treatment 1 / Date...

Treatment 2 / Date...

Treatment 3 / Date...

Treatment 4 / Date...

AFTERCARE AND GENERAL ADVICE

Treatment 1...

Treatment 2 ....

Treatment 3 ....

Treatment 4 ....

CLIENT'S FEEDBACK/ COMMENTS

Signature .... Date...

INDIAN HEAD MASSAGE CONSULTATION FORM

Therapist:	Therapist's address:	Date:
Client's name	Age	Gender
Client's address: Tel No:	Occupation:	Doctor's address/Telephone No. :

CONTRA-INDICATIONS

Diabetes	Cuts / Abrasions/recent scars	Spastic conditions
Abnormal blood pressure	Migraine	Sties
Epilepsy	Osteoporosis	Conjunctivitis
Cancer	Local infections	Advanced asthma
Undiagnosed lumps	Contagious skin disorders	Herpes Simplex
Thrombosis / Embolism	Fractures / Sprains	Other

CAUTIONS

Thrombosis/Strokes	Osteoporosis	Back/Neck problems
Aneurosa	Spondilitis	Recent operations
M.E.	Thyroid problems	Medication taken

LIFESTYLE / OTHER DETAILS

Occupation		Sleep patterns	
General Health		Allergies	
Exercise		Medication taken	
Diet		History of headaches/ migraines	
Fluid intake (water,		Emotional /	

juice)		psychological state at present	
Smoking		Stress levels	
Alcohol		Methods of relaxation	

OBJECTIVES OF THE TREATMENT & TREATMENT PLAN

What does the client hope to achieve?	
What will it be possible to achieve realistically? (Short term and long-term goals)	
Treatment plan agreed with the client (number of treatments to be given, over what period of time, length of time between treatments, areas to be paid particular attention to during the treatments)	

DISCLAIMER

I declare, that all the information regarding me in this form is true and accurate, and as far as I am aware, I can undertake a massage treatment without any adverse effects. I have been fully informed of any contra-indications and I am willing to undertake the treatment with this therapist.

Client's signature..Date...

TREATMENT DETAILS & CLIENT RESPONSE TO TREATMENT

Medium used:

Treatment 1 / Date...

Treatment 2 / Date...

Treatment 3 / Date...

Treatment 4 / Date...

Client's response / reactions to the treatments:

Treatment 1 / Date..

Treatment 2 / Date..

Treatment 3 / Date..

Treatment 4 / Date..

AFTERCARE AND GENERAL ADVICE

Treatment 1..

Treatment 2 ....

Treatment 3 ....

Treatment 4 ....

CLIENT'S FEEDBACK/ COMMENTS

Signature .... Date...

INDIAN HEAD MASSAGE CONSULTATION FORM

Therapist:	Therapist's address:	Date:
Client's name	Age	Gender
Client's address: Tel No:	Occupation:	Doctor's address/Telephone No. :

CONTRA-INDICATIONS

Diabetes	Cuts / Abrasions/recent scars	Spastic conditions
Abnormal blood pressure	Migraine	Sties
Epilepsy	Osteoporosis	Conjunctivitis
Cancer	Local infections	Advanced asthma
Undiagnosed lumps	Contagious skin disorders	Herpes Simplex
Thrombosis / Embolism	Fractures / Sprains	Other

CAUTIONS

Thrombosis/Strokes	Osteoporosis	Back/Neck problems
Aneurosa	Spondilitis	Recent operations
M.E.	Thyroid problems	Medication taken

LIFESTYLE / OTHER DETAILS

Occupation		Sleep patterns	
General Health		Allergies	
Exercise		Medication taken	
Diet		History of headaches/ migraines	
Fluid intake (water,		Emotional /	

juice)		psychological state at present	
Smoking		Stress levels	
Alcohol		Methods of relaxation	

OBJECTIVES OF THE TREATMENT & TREATMENT PLAN

What does the client hope to achieve?	
What will it be possible to achieve realistically? (Short term and long-term goals)	
Treatment plan agreed with the client (number of treatments to be given, over what period of time, length of time between treatments, areas to be paid particular attention to during the treatments)	

DISCLAIMER

I declare, that all the information regarding me in this form is true and accurate, and as far as I am aware, I can undertake a massage treatment without any adverse effects. I have been fully informed of any contra-indications and I am willing to undertake the treatment with this therapist.

Client's signature...Date...

TREATMENT DETAILS & CLIENT RESPONSE TO TREATMENT

Medium used:

Treatment 1 / Date...

Treatment 2 / Date...

Treatment 3 / Date...

Treatment 4 / Date...

Client's response / reactions to the treatments:

Treatment 1 / Date...

Treatment 2 / Date...

Treatment 3 / Date...

Treatment 4 / Date...

AFTERCARE AND GENERAL ADVICE

Treatment 1...

Treatment 2 ....

Treatment 3 ....

Treatment 4 ....

CLIENT'S FEEDBACK/ COMMENTS

Signature .... Date...

INDIAN HEAD MASSAGE CONSULTATION FORM

Therapist:	Therapist's address:	Date:
Client's name	Age	Gender
Client's address: Tel No:	Occupation:	Doctor's address/Telephone No. :

CONTRA-INDICATIONS

Diabetes	Cuts / Abrasions/recent scars	Spastic conditions
Abnormal blood pressure	Migraine	Sties
Epilepsy	Osteoporosis	Conjunctivitis
Cancer	Local infections	Advanced asthma
Undiagnosed lumps	Contagious skin disorders	Herpes Simplex
Thrombosis / Embolism	Fractures / Sprains	Other

CAUTIONS

Thrombosis/Strokes	Osteoporosis	Back/Neck problems
Aneurosa	Spondilitis	Recent operations
M.E.	Thyroid problems	Medication taken

LIFESTYLE / OTHER DETAILS

Occupation		Sleep patterns	
General Health		Allergies	
Exercise		Medication taken	
Diet		History of headaches/ migraines	
Fluid intake (water,		Emotional /	

juice)		psychological state at present	
Smoking		Stress levels	
Alcohol		Methods of relaxation	

OBJECTIVES OF THE TREATMENT & TREATMENT PLAN

What does the client hope to achieve?	
What will it be possible to achieve realistically? (Short term and long-term goals)	
Treatment plan agreed with the client (number of treatments to be given, over what period of time, length of time between treatments, areas to be paid particular attention to during the treatments)	

DISCLAIMER

I declare, that all the information regarding me in this form is true and accurate, and as far as I am aware, I can undertake a massage treatment without any adverse effects. I have been fully informed of any contra-indications and I am willing to undertake the treatment with this therapist.

Client's signature..Date...

TREATMENT DETAILS & CLIENT RESPONSE TO TREATMENT

Medium used:

Treatment 1 / Date..

Treatment 2 / Date..

Treatment 3 / Date..

Treatment 4 / Date..

Client's response / reactions to the treatments:

Treatment 1 / Date..

Treatment 2 / Date..

Treatment 3 / Date..

Treatment 4 / Date..

AFTERCARE AND GENERAL ADVICE

Treatment 1..

Treatment 2..

Treatment 3..

Treatment 4..

CLIENT'S FEEDBACK/ COMMENTS

Signature .... Date...

INDIAN HEAD MASSAGE CONSULTATION FORM

Therapist:	Therapist's address:	Date:
Client's name	Age	Gender
Client's address: Tel No:	Occupation:	Doctor's address/Telephone No. :

CONTRA-INDICATIONS

Diabetes	Cuts / Abrasions/recent scars	Spastic conditions
Abnormal blood pressure	Migraine	Sties
Epilepsy	Osteoporosis	Conjunctivitis
Cancer	Local infections	Advanced asthma
Undiagnosed lumps	Contagious skin disorders	Herpes Simplex
Thrombosis / Embolism	Fractures / Sprains	Other

CAUTIONS

Thrombosis/Strokes	Osteoporosis	Back/Neck problems
Aneurosa	Spondilitis	Recent operations
M.E.	Thyroid problems	Medication taken

LIFESTYLE / OTHER DETAILS

Occupation		Sleep patterns	
General Health		Allergies	
Exercise		Medication taken	
Diet		History of headaches/ migraines	
Fluid intake (water,		Emotional /	

juice)		psychological state at present	
Smoking		Stress levels	
Alcohol		Methods of relaxation	

OBJECTIVES OF THE TREATMENT & TREATMENT PLAN

What does the client hope to achieve?	
What will it be possible to achieve realistically? (Short term and long-term goals)	
Treatment plan agreed with the client (number of treatments to be given, over what period of time, length of time between treatments, areas to be paid particular attention to during the treatments)	

DISCLAIMER

I declare, that all the information regarding me in this form is true and accurate, and as far as I am aware, I can undertake a massage treatment without any adverse effects. I have been fully informed of any contra-indications and I am willing to undertake the treatment with this therapist.

Client's signature...Date..

TREATMENT DETAILS & CLIENT RESPONSE TO TREATMENT

Medium used:

Treatment 1 / Date...

Treatment 2 / Date...

Treatment 3 / Date...

Treatment 4 / Date...

Client's response / reactions to the treatments:

Treatment 1 / Date...

Treatment 2 / Date..

Treatment 3 / Date..

Treatment 4 / Date...

AFTERCARE AND GENERAL ADVICE

Treatment 1...

Treatment 2 ....

Treatment 3 ....

Treatment 4 ....

CLIENT'S FEEDBACK/ COMMENTS

Signature .... Date..

INDIAN HEAD MASSAGE CONSULTATION FORM

Therapist:	Therapist's address:	Date:
Client's name	Age	Gender
Client's address: Tel No:	Occupation:	Doctor's address/Telephone No. :

CONTRA-INDICATIONS

Diabetes	Cuts / Abrasions/recent scars	Spastic conditions
Abnormal blood pressure	Migraine	Sties
Epilepsy	Osteoporosis	Conjunctivitis
Cancer	Local infections	Advanced asthma
Undiagnosed lumps	Contagious skin disorders	Herpes Simplex
Thrombosis / Embolism	Fractures / Sprains	Other

CAUTIONS

Thrombosis/Strokes	Osteoporosis	Back/Neck problems
Aneurosa	Spondilitis	Recent operations
M.E.	Thyroid problems	Medication taken

LIFESTYLE / OTHER DETAILS

Occupation		Sleep patterns	
General Health		Allergies	
Exercise		Medication taken	
Diet		History of headaches/ migraines	
Fluid intake (water,		Emotional /	

juice)		psychological state at present	
Smoking		Stress levels	
Alcohol		Methods of relaxation	

OBJECTIVES OF THE TREATMENT & TREATMENT PLAN

What does the client hope to achieve?	
What will it be possible to achieve realistically? (Short term and long-term goals)	
Treatment plan agreed with the client (number of treatments to be given, over what period of time, length of time between treatments, areas to be paid particular attention to during the treatments)	

DISCLAIMER

I declare, that all the information regarding me in this form is true and accurate, and as far as I am aware, I can undertake a massage treatment without any adverse effects. I have been fully informed of any contra-indications and I am willing to undertake the treatment with this therapist.

Client's signature...Date...

TREATMENT DETAILS & CLIENT RESPONSE TO TREATMENT

Medium used:

Treatment 1 / Date..

Treatment 2 / Date..

Treatment 3 / Date..

Treatment 4 / Date..

Client's response / reactions to the treatments:

Treatment 1 / Date...

Treatment 2 / Date...

Treatment 3 / Date...

Treatment 4 / Date...

AFTERCARE AND GENERAL ADVICE

Treatment 1...

Treatment 2 ....

Treatment 3 ....

Treatment 4 ....

CLIENT'S FEEDBACK/ COMMENTS

Signature .... Date...

INDIAN HEAD MASSAGE CONSULTATION FORM

Therapist:	Therapist's address:	Date:
Client's name	Age	Gender
Client's address: Tel No:	Occupation:	Doctor's address/Telephone No. :

CONTRA-INDICATIONS

Diabetes	Cuts / Abrasions/recent scars	Spastic conditions
Abnormal blood pressure	Migraine	Sties
Epilepsy	Osteoporosis	Conjunctivitis
Cancer	Local infections	Advanced asthma
Undiagnosed lumps	Contagious skin disorders	Herpes Simplex
Thrombosis / Embolism	Fractures / Sprains	Other

CAUTIONS

Thrombosis/Strokes	Osteoporosis	Back/Neck problems
Aneurosa	Spondilitis	Recent operations
M.E.	Thyroid problems	Medication taken

LIFESTYLE / OTHER DETAILS

Occupation		Sleep patterns	
General Health		Allergies	
Exercise		Medication taken	
Diet		History of headaches/ migraines	
Fluid intake (water,		Emotional /	

juice)		psychological state at present	
Smoking		Stress levels	
Alcohol		Methods of relaxation	

OBJECTIVES OF THE TREATMENT & TREATMENT PLAN

What does the client hope to achieve?	
What will it be possible to achieve realistically? (Short term and long-term goals)	
Treatment plan agreed with the client (number of treatments to be given, over what period of time, length of time between treatments, areas to be paid particular attention to during the treatments)	

DISCLAIMER

I declare, that all the information regarding me in this form is true and accurate, and as far as I am aware, I can undertake a massage treatment without any adverse effects. I have been fully informed of any contra-indications and I am willing to undertake the treatment with this therapist.

Client's signature...Date..

TREATMENT DETAILS & CLIENT RESPONSE TO TREATMENT

Medium used:

Treatment 1 / Date...

Treatment 2 / Date...

Treatment 3 / Date...

Treatment 4 / Date...

Client's response / reactions to the treatments:

Treatment 1 / Date...

Treatment 2 / Date...

Treatment 3 / Date...

Treatment 4 / Date...

AFTERCARE AND GENERAL ADVICE

Treatment 1...

Treatment 2 ....

Treatment 3 ....

Treatment 4 ....

CLIENT'S FEEDBACK/ COMMENTS

Signature .... Date...

INDIAN HEAD MASSAGE CONSULTATION FORM

Therapist:	Therapist's address:	Date:
Client's name	Age	Gender
Client's address: Tel No:	Occupation:	Doctor's address/Telephone No. :

CONTRA-INDICATIONS

Diabetes	Cuts / Abrasions/recent scars	Spastic conditions
Abnormal blood pressure	Migraine	Sties
Epilepsy	Osteoporosis	Conjunctivitis
Cancer	Local infections	Advanced asthma
Undiagnosed lumps	Contagious skin disorders	Herpes Simplex
Thrombosis / Embolism	Fractures / Sprains	Other

CAUTIONS

Thrombosis/Strokes	Osteoporosis	Back/Neck problems
Aneurosa	Spondilitis	Recent operations
M.E.	Thyroid problems	Medication taken

LIFESTYLE / OTHER DETAILS

Occupation		Sleep patterns	
General Health		Allergies	
Exercise		Medication taken	
Diet		History of headaches/ migraines	
Fluid intake (water,		Emotional /	

juice)		psychological state at present	
Smoking		Stress levels	
Alcohol		Methods of relaxation	

OBJECTIVES OF THE TREATMENT & TREATMENT PLAN

What does the client hope to achieve?	
What will it be possible to achieve realistically? (Short term and long-term goals)	
Treatment plan agreed with the client (number of treatments to be given, over what period of time, length of time between treatments, areas to be paid particular attention to during the treatments)	

DISCLAIMER

I declare, that all the information regarding me in this form is true and accurate, and as far as I am aware, I can undertake a massage treatment without any adverse effects. I have been fully informed of any contra-indications and I am willing to undertake the treatment with this therapist.

Client's signature...Date...

TREATMENT DETAILS & CLIENT RESPONSE TO TREATMENT

Medium used:

Treatment 1 / Date...

Treatment 2 / Date...

Treatment 3 / Date...

Treatment 4 / Date...

Client's response / reactions to the treatments:

Treatment 1 / Date...

Treatment 2 / Date..

Treatment 3 / Date...

Treatment 4 / Date...

AFTERCARE AND GENERAL ADVICE

Treatment 1...

Treatment 2 ....

Treatment 3 ....

Treatment 4 ....

CLIENT'S FEEDBACK/ COMMENTS

Signature .... Date...

INDIAN HEAD MASSAGE CONSULTATION FORM

Therapist:	Therapist's address:	Date:
Client's name	Age	Gender
Client's address: Tel No:	Occupation:	Doctor's address/Telephone No. :

CONTRA-INDICATIONS

Diabetes	Cuts / Abrasions/recent scars	Spastic conditions
Abnormal blood pressure	Migraine	Sties
Epilepsy	Osteoporosis	Conjunctivitis
Cancer	Local infections	Advanced asthma
Undiagnosed lumps	Contagious skin disorders	Herpes Simplex
Thrombosis / Embolism	Fractures / Sprains	Other

CAUTIONS

Thrombosis/Strokes	Osteoporosis	Back/Neck problems
Aneurosa	Spondilitis	Recent operations
M.E.	Thyroid problems	Medication taken

LIFESTYLE / OTHER DETAILS

Occupation		Sleep patterns	
General Health		Allergies	
Exercise		Medication taken	
Diet		History of headaches/ migraines	
Fluid intake (water,		Emotional /	

juice)		psychological state at present	
Smoking		Stress levels	
Alcohol		Methods of relaxation	

OBJECTIVES OF THE TREATMENT & TREATMENT PLAN

What does the client hope to achieve?	
What will it be possible to achieve realistically? (Short term and long-term goals)	
Treatment plan agreed with the client (number of treatments to be given, over what period of time, length of time between treatments, areas to be paid particular attention to during the treatments)	

DISCLAIMER

I declare, that all the information regarding me in this form is true and accurate, and as far as I am aware, I can undertake a massage treatment without any adverse effects. I have been fully informed of any contra-indications and I am willing to undertake the treatment with this therapist.

Client's signature...Date...

TREATMENT DETAILS & CLIENT RESPONSE TO TREATMENT

Medium used:

Treatment 1 / Date...

Treatment 2 / Date...

Treatment 3 / Date...

Treatment 4 / Date...

Client's response / reactions to the treatments:

Treatment 1 / Date..

Treatment 2 / Date..

Treatment 3 / Date..

Treatment 4 / Date..

AFTERCARE AND GENERAL ADVICE

Treatment 1..

Treatment 2..

Treatment 3..

Treatment 4..

CLIENT'S FEEDBACK/ COMMENTS

Signature .... Date..

INDIAN HEAD MASSAGE CONSULTATION FORM

Therapist:	Therapist's address:	Date:
Client's name	Age	Gender
Client's address: Tel No:	Occupation:	Doctor's address/Telephone No. :

CONTRA-INDICATIONS

Diabetes	Cuts / Abrasions/recent scars	Spastic conditions
Abnormal blood pressure	Migraine	Sties
Epilepsy	Osteoporosis	Conjunctivitis
Cancer	Local infections	Advanced asthma
Undiagnosed lumps	Contagious skin disorders	Herpes Simplex
Thrombosis / Embolism	Fractures / Sprains	Other

CAUTIONS

Thrombosis/Strokes	Osteoporosis	Back/Neck problems
Aneurosa	Spondilitis	Recent operations
M.E.	Thyroid problems	Medication taken

LIFESTYLE / OTHER DETAILS

Occupation		Sleep patterns	
General Health		Allergies	
Exercise		Medication taken	
Diet		History of headaches/ migraines	
Fluid intake (water,		Emotional /	

juice)		psychological state at present	
Smoking		Stress levels	
Alcohol		Methods of relaxation	

OBJECTIVES OF THE TREATMENT & TREATMENT PLAN

What does the client hope to achieve?	
What will it be possible to achieve realistically? (Short term and long-term goals)	
Treatment plan agreed with the client (number of treatments to be given, over what period of time, length of time between treatments, areas to be paid particular attention to during the treatments)	

DISCLAIMER

I declare, that all the information regarding me in this form is true and accurate, and as far as I am aware, I can undertake a massage treatment without any adverse effects. I have been fully informed of any contra-indications and I am willing to undertake the treatment with this therapist.

Client's signature...Date...

TREATMENT DETAILS & CLIENT RESPONSE TO TREATMENT

Medium used:

Treatment 1 / Date...

Treatment 2 / Date...

Treatment 3 / Date...

Treatment 4 / Date...

Client's response / reactions to the treatments:

Treatment 1 / Date...

Treatment 2 / Date...

Treatment 3 / Date...

Treatment 4 / Date...

AFTERCARE AND GENERAL ADVICE

Treatment 1..

Treatment 2..

Treatment 3..

Treatment 4..

CLIENT'S FEEDBACK/ COMMENTS

Signature .... Date...

INDIAN HEAD MASSAGE CONSULTATION FORM

Therapist:	Therapist's address:	Date:
Client's name	Age	Gender
Client's address: Tel No:	Occupation:	Doctor's address/Telephone No. :

CONTRA-INDICATIONS

Diabetes	Cuts / Abrasions/recent scars	Spastic conditions
Abnormal blood pressure	Migraine	Sties
Epilepsy	Osteoporosis	Conjunctivitis
Cancer	Local infections	Advanced asthma
Undiagnosed lumps	Contagious skin disorders	Herpes Simplex
Thrombosis / Embolism	Fractures / Sprains	Other

CAUTIONS

Thrombosis/Strokes	Osteoporosis	Back/Neck problems
Aneurosa	Spondilitis	Recent operations
M.E.	Thyroid problems	Medication taken

LIFESTYLE / OTHER DETAILS

Occupation		Sleep patterns	
General Health		Allergies	
Exercise		Medication taken	
Diet		History of headaches/ migraines	
Fluid intake (water,		Emotional /	

juice)		psychological state at present	
Smoking		Stress levels	
Alcohol		Methods of relaxation	

OBJECTIVES OF THE TREATMENT & TREATMENT PLAN

What does the client hope to achieve?	
What will it be possible to achieve realistically? (Short term and long-term goals)	
Treatment plan agreed with the client (number of treatments to be given, over what period of time, length of time between treatments, areas to be paid particular attention to during the treatments)	

DISCLAIMER

I declare, that all the information regarding me in this form is true and accurate, and as far as I am aware, I can undertake a massage treatment without any adverse effects. I have been fully informed of any contra-indications and I am willing to undertake the treatment with this therapist.

Client's signature..Date..

TREATMENT DETAILS & CLIENT RESPONSE TO TREATMENT

Medium used:

Treatment 1 / Date...

Treatment 2 / Date...

Treatment 3 / Date...

Treatment 4 / Date...

Client's response / reactions to the treatments:

Treatment 1 / Date..

Treatment 2 / Date..

Treatment 3 / Date..

Treatment 4 / Date..

AFTERCARE AND GENERAL ADVICE

Treatment 1...

Treatment 2 ....

Treatment 3 ....

Treatment 4 ....

CLIENT'S FEEDBACK/ COMMENTS

Signature .... Date..

INDIAN HEAD MASSAGE CONSULTATION FORM

Therapist:	Therapist's address:	Date:
Client's name	Age	Gender
Client's address: Tel No:	Occupation:	Doctor's address/Telephone No. :

CONTRA-INDICATIONS

Diabetes	Cuts / Abrasions/recent scars	Spastic conditions
Abnormal blood pressure	Migraine	Sties
Epilepsy	Osteoporosis	Conjunctivitis
Cancer	Local infections	Advanced asthma
Undiagnosed lumps	Contagious skin disorders	Herpes Simplex
Thrombosis / Embolism	Fractures / Sprains	Other

CAUTIONS

Thrombosis/Strokes	Osteoporosis	Back/Neck problems
Aneurosa	Spondilitis	Recent operations
M.E.	Thyroid problems	Medication taken

LIFESTYLE / OTHER DETAILS

Occupation		Sleep patterns	
General Health		Allergies	
Exercise		Medication taken	
Diet		History of headaches/ migraines	
Fluid intake (water,		Emotional /	

juice)		psychological state at present	
Smoking		Stress levels	
Alcohol		Methods of relaxation	

OBJECTIVES OF THE TREATMENT & TREATMENT PLAN

What does the client hope to achieve?	
What will it be possible to achieve realistically? (Short term and long-term goals)	
Treatment plan agreed with the client (number of treatments to be given, over what period of time, length of time between treatments, areas to be paid particular attention to during the treatments)	

DISCLAIMER

I declare, that all the information regarding me in this form is true and accurate, and as far as I am aware, I can undertake a massage treatment without any adverse effects. I have been fully informed of any contra-indications and I am willing to undertake the treatment with this therapist.

Client's signature...Date...

TREATMENT DETAILS & CLIENT RESPONSE TO TREATMENT

Medium used:
Treatment 1 / Date..
Treatment 2 / Date..
Treatment 3 / Date..
Treatment 4 / Date..

Client's response / reactions to the treatments:

Treatment 1 / Date..

Treatment 2 / Date..

Treatment 3 / Date..

Treatment 4 / Date..

AFTERCARE AND GENERAL ADVICE

Treatment 1...

Treatment 2 ....

Treatment 3 ....

Treatment 4 ....

CLIENT'S FEEDBACK/ COMMENTS

Signature .... Date...

INDIAN HEAD MASSAGE CONSULTATION FORM

Therapist:	Therapist's address:	Date:
Client's name	Age	Gender
Client's address: Tel No:	Occupation:	Doctor's address/Telephone No. :

CONTRA-INDICATIONS

Diabetes	Cuts / Abrasions/recent scars	Spastic conditions
Abnormal blood pressure	Migraine	Sties
Epilepsy	Osteoporosis	Conjunctivitis
Cancer	Local infections	Advanced asthma
Undiagnosed lumps	Contagious skin disorders	Herpes Simplex
Thrombosis / Embolism	Fractures / Sprains	Other

CAUTIONS

Thrombosis/Strokes	Osteoporosis	Back/Neck problems
Aneurosa	Spondilitis	Recent operations
M.E.	Thyroid problems	Medication taken

LIFESTYLE / OTHER DETAILS

Occupation		Sleep patterns	
General Health		Allergies	
Exercise		Medication taken	
Diet		History of headaches/ migraines	
Fluid intake (water,		Emotional /	

juice)		psychological state at present	
Smoking		Stress levels	
Alcohol		Methods of relaxation	

OBJECTIVES OF THE TREATMENT & TREATMENT PLAN

What does the client hope to achieve?	
What will it be possible to achieve realistically? (Short term and long-term goals)	
Treatment plan agreed with the client (number of treatments to be given, over what period of time, length of time between treatments, areas to be paid particular attention to during the treatments)	

DISCLAIMER

I declare, that all the information regarding me in this form is true and accurate, and as far as I am aware, I can undertake a massage treatment without any adverse effects. I have been fully informed of any contra-indications and I am willing to undertake the treatment with this therapist.

Client's signature..Date...

TREATMENT DETAILS & CLIENT RESPONSE TO TREATMENT

Medium used:

Treatment 1 / Date...

Treatment 2 / Date...

Treatment 3 / Date...

Treatment 4 / Date...

Client's response / reactions to the treatments:

Treatment 1 / Date..

Treatment 2 / Date..

Treatment 3 / Date..

Treatment 4 / Date..

AFTERCARE AND GENERAL ADVICE

Treatment 1..

Treatment 2 ....

Treatment 3 ....

Treatment 4 ....

CLIENT'S FEEDBACK/ COMMENTS

Signature .... Date..

INDIAN HEAD MASSAGE CONSULTATION FORM

Therapist:	Therapist's address:	Date:
Client's name	Age	Gender
Client's address: Tel No:	Occupation:	Doctor's address/Telephone No. :

CONTRA-INDICATIONS

Diabetes	Cuts / Abrasions/recent scars	Spastic conditions
Abnormal blood pressure	Migraine	Sties
Epilepsy	Osteoporosis	Conjunctivitis
Cancer	Local infections	Advanced asthma
Undiagnosed lumps	Contagious skin disorders	Herpes Simplex
Thrombosis / Embolism	Fractures / Sprains	Other

CAUTIONS

Thrombosis/Strokes	Osteoporosis	Back/Neck problems
Aneurosa	Spondilitis	Recent operations
M.E.	Thyroid problems	Medication taken

LIFESTYLE / OTHER DETAILS

Occupation		Sleep patterns	
General Health		Allergies	
Exercise		Medication taken	
Diet		History of headaches/ migraines	
Fluid intake (water,		Emotional /	

juice)		psychological state at present	
Smoking		Stress levels	
Alcohol		Methods of relaxation	

OBJECTIVES OF THE TREATMENT & TREATMENT PLAN

What does the client hope to achieve?	
What will it be possible to achieve realistically? (Short term and long-term goals)	
Treatment plan agreed with the client (number of treatments to be given, over what period of time, length of time between treatments, areas to be paid particular attention to during the treatments)	

DISCLAIMER

I declare, that all the information regarding me in this form is true and accurate, and as far as I am aware, I can undertake a massage treatment without any adverse effects. I have been fully informed of any contra-indications and I am willing to undertake the treatment with this therapist.

Client's signature...Date...

TREATMENT DETAILS & CLIENT RESPONSE TO TREATMENT

Medium used:

Treatment 1 / Date..

Treatment 2 / Date..

Treatment 3 / Date..

Treatment 4 / Date..

Client's response / reactions to the treatments:

Treatment 1 / Date..

Treatment 2 / Date..

Treatment 3 / Date..

Treatment 4 / Date...

AFTERCARE AND GENERAL ADVICE

Treatment 1...

Treatment 2 ....

Treatment 3 ....

Treatment 4 ....

CLIENT'S FEEDBACK/ COMMENTS

Signature .... Date...

INDIAN HEAD MASSAGE CONSULTATION FORM

Therapist:	Therapist's address:	Date:
Client's name	Age	Gender
Client's address: Tel No:	Occupation:	Doctor's address/Telephone No. :

CONTRA-INDICATIONS

Diabetes	Cuts / Abrasions/recent scars	Spastic conditions
Abnormal blood pressure	Migraine	Sties
Epilepsy	Osteoporosis	Conjunctivitis
Cancer	Local infections	Advanced asthma
Undiagnosed lumps	Contagious skin disorders	Herpes Simplex
Thrombosis / Embolism	Fractures / Sprains	Other

CAUTIONS

Thrombosis/Strokes	Osteoporosis	Back/Neck problems
Aneurosa	Spondilitis	Recent operations
M.E.	Thyroid problems	Medication taken

LIFESTYLE / OTHER DETAILS

Occupation		Sleep patterns	
General Health		Allergies	
Exercise		Medication taken	
Diet		History of headaches/ migraines	
Fluid intake (water,		Emotional /	

juice)		psychological state at present	
Smoking		Stress levels	
Alcohol		Methods of relaxation	

OBJECTIVES OF THE TREATMENT & TREATMENT PLAN

What does the client hope to achieve?	
What will it be possible to achieve realistically? (Short term and long-term goals)	
Treatment plan agreed with the client (number of treatments to be given, over what period of time, length of time between treatments, areas to be paid particular attention to during the treatments)	

DISCLAIMER

I declare, that all the information regarding me in this form is true and accurate, and as far as I am aware, I can undertake a massage treatment without any adverse effects. I have been fully informed of any contra-indications and I am willing to undertake the treatment with this therapist.

Client's signature...Date...

TREATMENT DETAILS & CLIENT RESPONSE TO TREATMENT

Medium used:

Treatment 1 / Date..

Treatment 2 / Date..

Treatment 3 / Date..

Treatment 4 / Date..

Client's response / reactions to the treatments:

Treatment 1 / Date..

Treatment 2 / Date..

Treatment 3 / Date..

Treatment 4 / Date..

AFTERCARE AND GENERAL ADVICE

Treatment 1..

Treatment 2 ....

Treatment 3 ....

Treatment 4 ....

CLIENT'S FEEDBACK/ COMMENTS

Signature .... Date..

INDIAN HEAD MASSAGE CONSULTATION FORM

Therapist:	Therapist's address:	Date:
Client's name	Age	Gender
Client's address: Tel No:	Occupation:	Doctor's address/Telephone No. :

CONTRA-INDICATIONS

Diabetes	Cuts / Abrasions/recent scars	Spastic conditions
Abnormal blood pressure	Migraine	Sties
Epilepsy	Osteoporosis	Conjunctivitis
Cancer	Local infections	Advanced asthma
Undiagnosed lumps	Contagious skin disorders	Herpes Simplex
Thrombosis / Embolism	Fractures / Sprains	Other

CAUTIONS

Thrombosis/Strokes	Osteoporosis	Back/Neck problems
Aneurosa	Spondilitis	Recent operations
M.E.	Thyroid problems	Medication taken

LIFESTYLE / OTHER DETAILS

Occupation		Sleep patterns	
General Health		Allergies	
Exercise		Medication taken	
Diet		History of headaches/ migraines	
Fluid intake (water,		Emotional /	

juice)		psychological state at present	
Smoking		Stress levels	
Alcohol		Methods of relaxation	

OBJECTIVES OF THE TREATMENT & TREATMENT PLAN

What does the client hope to achieve?	
What will it be possible to achieve realistically? (Short term and long-term goals)	
Treatment plan agreed with the client (number of treatments to be given, over what period of time, length of time between treatments, areas to be paid particular attention to during the treatments)	

DISCLAIMER

I declare, that all the information regarding me in this form is true and accurate, and as far as I am aware, I can undertake a massage treatment without any adverse effects. I have been fully informed of any contra-indications and I am willing to undertake the treatment with this therapist.

Client's signature...Date..

TREATMENT DETAILS & CLIENT RESPONSE TO TREATMENT

Medium used:
Treatment 1 / Date...
Treatment 2 / Date...
Treatment 3 / Date...
Treatment 4 / Date...

Client's response / reactions to the treatments:

Treatment 1 / Date...

Treatment 2 / Date...

Treatment 3 / Date...

Treatment 4 / Date...

AFTERCARE AND GENERAL ADVICE

Treatment 1...

Treatment 2 ....

Treatment 3 ....

Treatment 4 ....

CLIENT'S FEEDBACK/ COMMENTS

Signature .... Date...

INDIAN HEAD MASSAGE CONSULTATION FORM

Therapist:	Therapist's address:	Date:
Client's name	Age	Gender
Client's address: Tel No:	Occupation:	Doctor's address/Telephone No. :

CONTRA-INDICATIONS

Diabetes	Cuts / Abrasions/recent scars	Spastic conditions
Abnormal blood pressure	Migraine	Sties
Epilepsy	Osteoporosis	Conjunctivitis
Cancer	Local infections	Advanced asthma
Undiagnosed lumps	Contagious skin disorders	Herpes Simplex
Thrombosis / Embolism	Fractures / Sprains	Other

CAUTIONS

Thrombosis/Strokes	Osteoporosis	Back/Neck problems
Aneurosa	Spondilitis	Recent operations
M.E.	Thyroid problems	Medication taken

LIFESTYLE / OTHER DETAILS

Occupation		Sleep patterns	
General Health		Allergies	
Exercise		Medication taken	
Diet		History of headaches/ migraines	
Fluid intake (water,		Emotional /	

juice)		psychological state at present	
Smoking		Stress levels	
Alcohol		Methods of relaxation	

OBJECTIVES OF THE TREATMENT & TREATMENT PLAN

What does the client hope to achieve?	
What will it be possible to achieve realistically? (Short term and long-term goals)	
Treatment plan agreed with the client (number of treatments to be given, over what period of time, length of time between treatments, areas to be paid particular attention to during the treatments)	

DISCLAIMER

I declare, that all the information regarding me in this form is true and accurate, and as far as I am aware, I can undertake a massage treatment without any adverse effects. I have been fully informed of any contra-indications and I am willing to undertake the treatment with this therapist.

Client's signature...Date...

TREATMENT DETAILS & CLIENT RESPONSE TO TREATMENT

Medium used:

Treatment 1 / Date...

Treatment 2 / Date...

Treatment 3 / Date...

Treatment 4 / Date...

Client's response / reactions to the treatments:

Treatment 1 / Date...

Treatment 2 / Date...

Treatment 3 / Date...

Treatment 4 / Date...

AFTERCARE AND GENERAL ADVICE

Treatment 1...

Treatment 2 ....

Treatment 3 ....

Treatment 4 ....

CLIENT'S FEEDBACK/ COMMENTS

Signature .... Date...

INDIAN HEAD MASSAGE CONSULTATION FORM

Therapist:	Therapist's address:	Date:
Client's name	Age	Gender
Client's address: Tel No:	Occupation:	Doctor's address/Telephone No. :

CONTRA-INDICATIONS

Diabetes	Cuts / Abrasions/recent scars	Spastic conditions
Abnormal blood pressure	Migraine	Sties
Epilepsy	Osteoporosis	Conjunctivitis
Cancer	Local infections	Advanced asthma
Undiagnosed lumps	Contagious skin disorders	Herpes Simplex
Thrombosis / Embolism	Fractures / Sprains	Other

CAUTIONS

Thrombosis/Strokes	Osteoporosis	Back/Neck problems
Aneurosa	Spondilitis	Recent operations
M.E.	Thyroid problems	Medication taken

LIFESTYLE / OTHER DETAILS

Occupation		Sleep patterns	
General Health		Allergies	
Exercise		Medication taken	
Diet		History of headaches/ migraines	
Fluid intake (water,		Emotional /	

juice)		psychological state at present	
Smoking		Stress levels	
Alcohol		Methods of relaxation	

OBJECTIVES OF THE TREATMENT & TREATMENT PLAN

What does the client hope to achieve?	
What will it be possible to achieve realistically? (Short term and long-term goals)	
Treatment plan agreed with the client (number of treatments to be given, over what period of time, length of time between treatments, areas to be paid particular attention to during the treatments)	

DISCLAIMER

I declare, that all the information regarding me in this form is true and accurate, and as far as I am aware, I can undertake a massage treatment without any adverse effects. I have been fully informed of any contra-indications and I am willing to undertake the treatment with this therapist.

Client's signature..Date..

TREATMENT DETAILS & CLIENT RESPONSE TO TREATMENT

Medium used:

Treatment 1 / Date...

Treatment 2 / Date...

Treatment 3 / Date...

Treatment 4 / Date...

Client's response / reactions to the treatments:

Treatment 1 / Date..

Treatment 2 / Date..

Treatment 3 / Date..

Treatment 4 / Date..

AFTERCARE AND GENERAL ADVICE

Treatment 1..

Treatment 2 ....

Treatment 3 ....

Treatment 4 ....

CLIENT'S FEEDBACK/ COMMENTS

Signature .... Date..

INDIAN HEAD MASSAGE CONSULTATION FORM

Therapist:	Therapist's address:	Date:
Client's name	Age	Gender
Client's address: Tel No:	Occupation:	Doctor's address/Telephone No. :

CONTRA-INDICATIONS

Diabetes	Cuts / Abrasions/recent scars	Spastic conditions
Abnormal blood pressure	Migraine	Sties
Epilepsy	Osteoporosis	Conjunctivitis
Cancer	Local infections	Advanced asthma
Undiagnosed lumps	Contagious skin disorders	Herpes Simplex
Thrombosis / Embolism	Fractures / Sprains	Other

CAUTIONS

Thrombosis/Strokes	Osteoporosis	Back/Neck problems
Aneurosa	Spondilitis	Recent operations
M.E.	Thyroid problems	Medication taken

LIFESTYLE / OTHER DETAILS

Occupation		Sleep patterns	
General Health		Allergies	
Exercise		Medication taken	
Diet		History of headaches/ migraines	
Fluid intake (water,		Emotional /	

juice)		psychological state at present	
Smoking		Stress levels	
Alcohol		Methods of relaxation	

OBJECTIVES OF THE TREATMENT & TREATMENT PLAN

What does the client hope to achieve?	
What will it be possible to achieve realistically? (Short term and long-term goals)	
Treatment plan agreed with the client (number of treatments to be given, over what period of time, length of time between treatments, areas to be paid particular attention to during the treatments)	

DISCLAIMER

I declare, that all the information regarding me in this form is true and accurate, and as far as I am aware, I can undertake a massage treatment without any adverse effects. I have been fully informed of any contra-indications and I am willing to undertake the treatment with this therapist.

Client's signature..Date...

TREATMENT DETAILS & CLIENT RESPONSE TO TREATMENT

Medium used:

Treatment 1 / Date..

Treatment 2 / Date..

Treatment 3 / Date..

Treatment 4 / Date..

Client's response / reactions to the treatments:

Treatment 1 / Date...

Treatment 2 / Date...

Treatment 3 / Date...

Treatment 4 / Date...

AFTERCARE AND GENERAL ADVICE

Treatment 1...

Treatment 2 ....

Treatment 3 ....

Treatment 4 ....

CLIENT'S FEEDBACK/ COMMENTS

Signature .... Date...

INDIAN HEAD MASSAGE CONSULTATION FORM

Therapist:	Therapist's address:	Date:
Client's name	Age	Gender
Client's address: Tel No:	Occupation:	Doctor's address/Telephone No. :

CONTRA-INDICATIONS

Diabetes	Cuts / Abrasions/recent scars	Spastic conditions
Abnormal blood pressure	Migraine	Sties
Epilepsy	Osteoporosis	Conjunctivitis
Cancer	Local infections	Advanced asthma
Undiagnosed lumps	Contagious skin disorders	Herpes Simplex
Thrombosis / Embolism	Fractures / Sprains	Other

CAUTIONS

Thrombosis/Strokes	Osteoporosis	Back/Neck problems
Aneurosa	Spondilitis	Recent operations
M.E.	Thyroid problems	Medication taken

LIFESTYLE / OTHER DETAILS

Occupation		Sleep patterns	
General Health		Allergies	
Exercise		Medication taken	
Diet		History of headaches/ migraines	
Fluid intake (water,		Emotional /	

juice)		psychological state at present	
Smoking		Stress levels	
Alcohol		Methods of relaxation	

OBJECTIVES OF THE TREATMENT & TREATMENT PLAN

What does the client hope to achieve?	
What will it be possible to achieve realistically? (Short term and long-term goals)	
Treatment plan agreed with the client (number of treatments to be given, over what period of time, length of time between treatments, areas to be paid particular attention to during the treatments)	

DISCLAIMER

I declare, that all the information regarding me in this form is true and accurate, and as far as I am aware, I can undertake a massage treatment without any adverse effects. I have been fully informed of any contra-indications and I am willing to undertake the treatment with this therapist.

Client's signature...Date..

TREATMENT DETAILS & CLIENT RESPONSE TO TREATMENT

Medium used:

Treatment 1 / Date..

Treatment 2 / Date..

Treatment 3 / Date..

Treatment 4 / Date..

Client's response / reactions to the treatments:

Treatment 1 / Date..

Treatment 2 / Date..

Treatment 3 / Date..

Treatment 4 / Date..

AFTERCARE AND GENERAL ADVICE

Treatment 1...

Treatment 2 ....

Treatment 3 ....

Treatment 4 ....

CLIENT'S FEEDBACK/ COMMENTS

Signature .... Date...

INDIAN HEAD MASSAGE CONSULTATION FORM

Therapist:	Therapist's address:	Date:
Client's name	Age	Gender
Client's address: Tel No:	Occupation:	Doctor's address/Telephone No. :

CONTRA-INDICATIONS

Diabetes	Cuts / Abrasions/recent scars	Spastic conditions
Abnormal blood pressure	Migraine	Sties
Epilepsy	Osteoporosis	Conjunctivitis
Cancer	Local infections	Advanced asthma
Undiagnosed lumps	Contagious skin disorders	Herpes Simplex
Thrombosis / Embolism	Fractures / Sprains	Other

CAUTIONS

Thrombosis/Strokes	Osteoporosis	Back/Neck problems
Aneurosa	Spondilitis	Recent operations
M.E.	Thyroid problems	Medication taken

LIFESTYLE / OTHER DETAILS

Occupation		Sleep patterns	
General Health		Allergies	
Exercise		Medication taken	
Diet		History of headaches/ migraines	
Fluid intake (water,		Emotional /	

juice)		psychological state at present	
Smoking		Stress levels	
Alcohol		Methods of relaxation	

OBJECTIVES OF THE TREATMENT & TREATMENT PLAN

What does the client hope to achieve?	
What will it be possible to achieve realistically? (Short term and long-term goals)	
Treatment plan agreed with the client (number of treatments to be given, over what period of time, length of time between treatments, areas to be paid particular attention to during the treatments)	

DISCLAIMER

I declare, that all the information regarding me in this form is true and accurate, and as far as I am aware, I can undertake a massage treatment without any adverse effects. I have been fully informed of any contra-indications and I am willing to undertake the treatment with this therapist.

Client's signature...Date...

TREATMENT DETAILS & CLIENT RESPONSE TO TREATMENT

Medium used:

Treatment 1 / Date...

Treatment 2 / Date...

Treatment 3 / Date...

Treatment 4 / Date...

Client's response / reactions to the treatments:

Treatment 1 / Date..

Treatment 2 / Date..

Treatment 3 / Date..

Treatment 4 / Date..

AFTERCARE AND GENERAL ADVICE

Treatment 1..

Treatment 2..

Treatment 3..

Treatment 4..

CLIENT'S FEEDBACK/ COMMENTS

Signature .... Date..

INDIAN HEAD MASSAGE CONSULTATION FORM

Therapist:	Therapist's address:	Date:
Client's name	Age	Gender
Client's address: Tel No:	Occupation:	Doctor's address/Telephone No. :

CONTRA-INDICATIONS

Diabetes	Cuts / Abrasions/recent scars	Spastic conditions
Abnormal blood pressure	Migraine	Sties
Epilepsy	Osteoporosis	Conjunctivitis
Cancer	Local infections	Advanced asthma
Undiagnosed lumps	Contagious skin disorders	Herpes Simplex
Thrombosis / Embolism	Fractures / Sprains	Other

CAUTIONS

Thrombosis/Strokes	Osteoporosis	Back/Neck problems
Aneurosa	Spondilitis	Recent operations
M.E.	Thyroid problems	Medication taken

LIFESTYLE / OTHER DETAILS

Occupation		Sleep patterns	
General Health		Allergies	
Exercise		Medication taken	
Diet		History of headaches/ migraines	
Fluid intake (water,		Emotional /	

juice)		psychological state at present	
Smoking		Stress levels	
Alcohol		Methods of relaxation	

OBJECTIVES OF THE TREATMENT & TREATMENT PLAN

What does the client hope to achieve?	
What will it be possible to achieve realistically? (Short term and long-term goals)	
Treatment plan agreed with the client (number of treatments to be given, over what period of time, length of time between treatments, areas to be paid particular attention to during the treatments)	

DISCLAIMER

I declare, that all the information regarding me in this form is true and accurate, and as far as I am aware, I can undertake a massage treatment without any adverse effects. I have been fully informed of any contra-indications and I am willing to undertake the treatment with this therapist.

Client's signature...Date...

TREATMENT DETAILS & CLIENT RESPONSE TO TREATMENT

Medium used:

Treatment 1 / Date..

Treatment 2 / Date..

Treatment 3 / Date..

Treatment 4 / Date..

Client's response / reactions to the treatments:

Treatment 1 / Date...

Treatment 2 / Date...

Treatment 3 / Date...

Treatment 4 / Date...

AFTERCARE AND GENERAL ADVICE

Treatment 1...

Treatment 2 ....

Treatment 3 ....

Treatment 4 ....

CLIENT'S FEEDBACK/ COMMENTS

Signature .... Date...

INDIAN HEAD MASSAGE CONSULTATION FORM

Therapist:	Therapist's address:	Date:
Client's name	Age	Gender
Client's address: Tel No:	Occupation:	Doctor's address/Telephone No. :

CONTRA-INDICATIONS

Diabetes	Cuts / Abrasions/recent scars	Spastic conditions
Abnormal blood pressure	Migraine	Sties
Epilepsy	Osteoporosis	Conjunctivitis
Cancer	Local infections	Advanced asthma
Undiagnosed lumps	Contagious skin disorders	Herpes Simplex
Thrombosis / Embolism	Fractures / Sprains	Other

CAUTIONS

Thrombosis/Strokes	Osteoporosis	Back/Neck problems
Aneurosa	Spondilitis	Recent operations
M.E.	Thyroid problems	Medication taken

LIFESTYLE / OTHER DETAILS

Occupation		Sleep patterns	
General Health		Allergies	
Exercise		Medication taken	
Diet		History of headaches/ migraines	
Fluid intake (water,		Emotional /	

juice)		psychological state at present	
Smoking		Stress levels	
Alcohol		Methods of relaxation	

OBJECTIVES OF THE TREATMENT & TREATMENT PLAN

What does the client hope to achieve?	
What will it be possible to achieve realistically? (Short term and long-term goals)	
Treatment plan agreed with the client (number of treatments to be given, over what period of time, length of time between treatments, areas to be paid particular attention to during the treatments)	

DISCLAIMER

I declare, that all the information regarding me in this form is true and accurate, and as far as I am aware, I can undertake a massage treatment without any adverse effects. I have been fully informed of any contra-indications and I am willing to undertake the treatment with this therapist.

Client's signature...Date...

TREATMENT DETAILS & CLIENT RESPONSE TO TREATMENT

Medium used:

Treatment 1 / Date...

Treatment 2 / Date...

Treatment 3 / Date...

Treatment 4 / Date...

Client's response / reactions to the treatments:

Treatment 1 / Date..

Treatment 2 / Date..

Treatment 3 / Date..

Treatment 4 / Date..

AFTERCARE AND GENERAL ADVICE

Treatment 1..

Treatment 2 ....:......

Treatment 3 ....

Treatment 4 ....

CLIENT'S FEEDBACK/ COMMENTS

Signature .... Date...

INDIAN HEAD MASSAGE CONSULTATION FORM

Therapist:	Therapist's address:	Date:
Client's name	Age	Gender
Client's address: Tel No:	Occupation:	Doctor's address/Telephone No. :

CONTRA-INDICATIONS

Diabetes	Cuts / Abrasions/recent scars	Spastic conditions
Abnormal blood pressure	Migraine	Sties
Epilepsy	Osteoporosis	Conjunctivitis
Cancer	Local infections	Advanced asthma
Undiagnosed lumps	Contagious skin disorders	Herpes Simplex
Thrombosis / Embolism	Fractures / Sprains	Other

CAUTIONS

Thrombosis/Strokes	Osteoporosis	Back/Neck problems
Aneurosa	Spondilitis	Recent operations
M.E.	Thyroid problems	Medication taken

LIFESTYLE / OTHER DETAILS

Occupation		Sleep patterns	
General Health		Allergies	
Exercise		Medication taken	
Diet		History of headaches/ migraines	
Fluid intake (water,		Emotional /	

juice)		psychological state at present	
Smoking		Stress levels	
Alcohol		Methods of relaxation	

OBJECTIVES OF THE TREATMENT & TREATMENT PLAN

What does the client hope to achieve?	
What will it be possible to achieve realistically? (Short term and long-term goals)	
Treatment plan agreed with the client (number of treatments to be given, over what period of time, length of time between treatments, areas to be paid particular attention to during the treatments)	

DISCLAIMER

I declare, that all the information regarding me in this form is true and accurate, and as far as I am aware, I can undertake a massage treatment without any adverse effects. I have been fully informed of any contra-indications and I am willing to undertake the treatment with this therapist.

Client's signature...Date...

TREATMENT DETAILS & CLIENT RESPONSE TO TREATMENT

Medium used:

Treatment 1 / Date...

Treatment 2 / Date...

Treatment 3 / Date...

Treatment 4 / Date...

Client's response / reactions to the treatments:

Treatment 1 / Date...

Treatment 2 / Date...

Treatment 3 / Date...

Treatment 4 / Date...

AFTERCARE AND GENERAL ADVICE

Treatment 1..

Treatment 2 ....

Treatment 3 ....

Treatment 4 ....

CLIENT'S FEEDBACK/ COMMENTS

Signature .... Date...

INDIAN HEAD MASSAGE CONSULTATION FORM

Therapist:	Therapist's address:	Date:
Client's name	Age	Gender
Client's address: Tel No:	Occupation:	Doctor's address/Telephone No. :

CONTRA-INDICATIONS

Diabetes	Cuts / Abrasions/recent scars	Spastic conditions
Abnormal blood pressure	Migraine	Sties
Epilepsy	Osteoporosis	Conjunctivitis
Cancer	Local infections	Advanced asthma
Undiagnosed lumps	Contagious skin disorders	Herpes Simplex
Thrombosis / Embolism	Fractures / Sprains	Other

CAUTIONS

Thrombosis/Strokes	Osteoporosis	Back/Neck problems
Aneurosa	Spondilitis	Recent operations
M.E.	Thyroid problems	Medication taken

LIFESTYLE / OTHER DETAILS

Occupation		Sleep patterns	
General Health		Allergies	
Exercise		Medication taken	
Diet		History of headaches/ migraines	
Fluid intake (water,		Emotional /	

juice)		psychological state at present	
Smoking		Stress levels	
Alcohol		Methods of relaxation	

OBJECTIVES OF THE TREATMENT & TREATMENT PLAN

What does the client hope to achieve?	
What will it be possible to achieve realistically? (Short term and long-term goals)	
Treatment plan agreed with the client (number of treatments to be given, over what period of time, length of time between treatments, areas to be paid particular attention to during the treatments)	

DISCLAIMER

I declare, that all the information regarding me in this form is true and accurate, and as far as I am aware, I can undertake a massage treatment without any adverse effects. I have been fully informed of any contra-indications and I am willing to undertake the treatment with this therapist.

Client's signature...Date...

TREATMENT DETAILS & CLIENT RESPONSE TO TREATMENT

Medium used:

Treatment 1 / Date..

Treatment 2 / Date..

Treatment 3 / Date..

Treatment 4 / Date..

Client's response / reactions to the treatments:

Treatment 1 / Date...

Treatment 2 / Date...

Treatment 3 / Date...

Treatment 4 / Date...

AFTERCARE AND GENERAL ADVICE

Treatment 1...

Treatment 2 ....

Treatment 3 ....

Treatment 4 ....

CLIENT'S FEEDBACK/ COMMENTS

Signature .... Date...

INDIAN HEAD MASSAGE CONSULTATION FORM

Therapist:	Therapist's address:	Date:
Client's name	Age	Gender
Client's address: Tel No:	Occupation:	Doctor's address/Telephone No. :

CONTRA-INDICATIONS

Diabetes	Cuts / Abrasions/recent scars	Spastic conditions
Abnormal blood pressure	Migraine	Sties
Epilepsy	Osteoporosis	Conjunctivitis
Cancer	Local infections	Advanced asthma
Undiagnosed lumps	Contagious skin disorders	Herpes Simplex
Thrombosis / Embolism	Fractures / Sprains	Other

CAUTIONS

Thrombosis/Strokes	Osteoporosis	Back/Neck problems
Aneurosa	Spondilitis	Recent operations
M.E.	Thyroid problems	Medication taken

LIFESTYLE / OTHER DETAILS

Occupation		Sleep patterns	
General Health		Allergies	
Exercise		Medication taken	
Diet		History of headaches/ migraines	
Fluid intake (water,		Emotional /	

juice)		psychological state at present	
Smoking		Stress levels	
Alcohol		Methods of relaxation	

OBJECTIVES OF THE TREATMENT & TREATMENT PLAN

What does the client hope to achieve?	
What will it be possible to achieve realistically? (Short term and long-term goals)	
Treatment plan agreed with the client (number of treatments to be given, over what period of time, length of time between treatments, areas to be paid particular attention to during the treatments)	

DISCLAIMER

I declare, that all the information regarding me in this form is true and accurate, and as far as I am aware, I can undertake a massage treatment without any adverse effects. I have been fully informed of any contra-indications and I am willing to undertake the treatment with this therapist.

Client's signature..Date..

TREATMENT DETAILS & CLIENT RESPONSE TO TREATMENT

Medium used:

Treatment 1 / Date..

Treatment 2 / Date..

Treatment 3 / Date..

Treatment 4 / Date..

Client's response / reactions to the treatments:

Treatment 1 / Date..

Treatment 2 / Date..

Treatment 3 / Date..

Treatment 4 / Date..

AFTERCARE AND GENERAL ADVICE

Treatment 1...

Treatment 2 ....

Treatment 3 ....

Treatment 4 ....

CLIENT'S FEEDBACK/ COMMENTS

Signature .... Date..

INDIAN HEAD MASSAGE CONSULTATION FORM

Therapist:	Therapist's address:	Date:
Client's name	Age	Gender
Client's address: Tel No:	Occupation:	Doctor's address/Telephone No. :

CONTRA-INDICATIONS

Diabetes	Cuts / Abrasions/recent scars	Spastic conditions
Abnormal blood pressure	Migraine	Sties
Epilepsy	Osteoporosis	Conjunctivitis
Cancer	Local infections	Advanced asthma
Undiagnosed lumps	Contagious skin disorders	Herpes Simplex
Thrombosis / Embolism	Fractures / Sprains	Other

CAUTIONS

Thrombosis/Strokes	Osteoporosis	Back/Neck problems
Aneurosa	Spondilitis	Recent operations
M.E.	Thyroid problems	Medication taken

LIFESTYLE / OTHER DETAILS

Occupation		Sleep patterns	
General Health		Allergies	
Exercise		Medication taken	
Diet		History of headaches/ migraines	
Fluid intake (water,		Emotional /	

juice)		psychological state at present	
Smoking		Stress levels	
Alcohol		Methods of relaxation	

OBJECTIVES OF THE TREATMENT & TREATMENT PLAN

What does the client hope to achieve?	
What will it be possible to achieve realistically? (Short term and long-term goals)	
Treatment plan agreed with the client (number of treatments to be given, over what period of time, length of time between treatments, areas to be paid particular attention to during the treatments)	

DISCLAIMER

I declare, that all the information regarding me in this form is true and accurate, and as far as I am aware, I can undertake a massage treatment without any adverse effects. I have been fully informed of any contra-indications and I am willing to undertake the treatment with this therapist.

Client's signature...Date..

TREATMENT DETAILS & CLIENT RESPONSE TO TREATMENT

Medium used:

Treatment 1 / Date...

Treatment 2 / Date...

Treatment 3 / Date...

Treatment 4 / Date...

Client's response / reactions to the treatments:

Treatment 1 / Date..

Treatment 2 / Date..

Treatment 3 / Date..

Treatment 4 / Date..

AFTERCARE AND GENERAL ADVICE

Treatment 1...

Treatment 2 ....

Treatment 3 ....

Treatment 4 ....

CLIENT'S FEEDBACK/ COMMENTS

Signature .... Date..

INDIAN HEAD MASSAGE CONSULTATION FORM

Therapist:	Therapist's address:	Date:
Client's name	Age	Gender
Client's address: Tel No:	Occupation:	Doctor's address/Telephone No. :

CONTRA-INDICATIONS

Diabetes	Cuts / Abrasions/recent scars	Spastic conditions
Abnormal blood pressure	Migraine	Sties
Epilepsy	Osteoporosis	Conjunctivitis
Cancer	Local infections	Advanced asthma
Undiagnosed lumps	Contagious skin disorders	Herpes Simplex
Thrombosis / Embolism	Fractures / Sprains	Other

CAUTIONS

Thrombosis/Strokes	Osteoporosis	Back/Neck problems
Aneurosa	Spondilitis	Recent operations
M.E.	Thyroid problems	Medication taken

LIFESTYLE / OTHER DETAILS

Occupation		Sleep patterns	
General Health		Allergies	
Exercise		Medication taken	
Diet		History of headaches/ migraines	
Fluid intake (water,		Emotional /	

juice)		psychological state at present	
Smoking		Stress levels	
Alcohol		Methods of relaxation	

OBJECTIVES OF THE TREATMENT & TREATMENT PLAN

What does the client hope to achieve?	
What will it be possible to achieve realistically? (Short term and long-term goals)	
Treatment plan agreed with the client (number of treatments to be given, over what period of time, length of time between treatments, areas to be paid particular attention to during the treatments)	

DISCLAIMER

I declare, that all the information regarding me in this form is true and accurate, and as far as I am aware, I can undertake a massage treatment without any adverse effects. I have been fully informed of any contra-indications and I am willing to undertake the treatment with this therapist.

Client's signature...Date...

TREATMENT DETAILS & CLIENT RESPONSE TO TREATMENT

Medium used:

Treatment 1 / Date...

Treatment 2 / Date...

Treatment 3 / Date...

Treatment 4 / Date...

Client's response / reactions to the treatments:

Treatment 1 / Date..

Treatment 2 / Date..

Treatment 3 / Date..

Treatment 4 / Date..

AFTERCARE AND GENERAL ADVICE

Treatment 1..

Treatment 2 ....

Treatment 3 ....

Treatment 4 ....

CLIENT'S FEEDBACK/ COMMENTS

Signature .... Date..

INDIAN HEAD MASSAGE CONSULTATION FORM

Therapist:	Therapist's address:	Date:
Client's name	Age	Gender
Client's address: Tel No:	Occupation:	Doctor's address/Telephone No. :

CONTRA-INDICATIONS

Diabetes	Cuts / Abrasions/recent scars	Spastic conditions
Abnormal blood pressure	Migraine	Sties
Epilepsy	Osteoporosis	Conjunctivitis
Cancer	Local infections	Advanced asthma
Undiagnosed lumps	Contagious skin disorders	Herpes Simplex
Thrombosis / Embolism	Fractures / Sprains	Other

CAUTIONS

Thrombosis/Strokes	Osteoporosis	Back/Neck problems
Aneurosa	Spondilitis	Recent operations
M.E.	Thyroid problems	Medication taken

LIFESTYLE / OTHER DETAILS

Occupation		Sleep patterns	
General Health		Allergies	
Exercise		Medication taken	
Diet		History of headaches/ migraines	
Fluid intake (water,		Emotional /	

juice)		psychological state at present	
Smoking		Stress levels	
Alcohol		Methods of relaxation	

OBJECTIVES OF THE TREATMENT & TREATMENT PLAN

What does the client hope to achieve?	
What will it be possible to achieve realistically? (Short term and long-term goals)	
Treatment plan agreed with the client (number of treatments to be given, over what period of time, length of time between treatments, areas to be paid particular attention to during the treatments)	

DISCLAIMER

I declare, that all the information regarding me in this form is true and accurate, and as far as I am aware, I can undertake a massage treatment without any adverse effects. I have been fully informed of any contra-indications and I am willing to undertake the treatment with this therapist.

Client's signature...Date...

TREATMENT DETAILS & CLIENT RESPONSE TO TREATMENT

Medium used:

Treatment 1 / Date...

Treatment 2 / Date...

Treatment 3 / Date...

Treatment 4 / Date...

Client's response / reactions to the treatments:

Treatment 1 / Date...

Treatment 2 / Date..

Treatment 3 / Date..

Treatment 4 / Date..

AFTERCARE AND GENERAL ADVICE

Treatment 1..

Treatment 2 ....

Treatment 3 ....

Treatment 4 ....

CLIENT'S FEEDBACK/ COMMENTS

Signature .... Date...

INDIAN HEAD MASSAGE CONSULTATION FORM

Therapist:	Therapist's address:	Date:
Client's name	Age	Gender
Client's address: Tel No:	Occupation:	Doctor's address/Telephone No. :

CONTRA-INDICATIONS

Diabetes	Cuts / Abrasions/recent scars	Spastic conditions
Abnormal blood pressure	Migraine	Sties
Epilepsy	Osteoporosis	Conjunctivitis
Cancer	Local infections	Advanced asthma
Undiagnosed lumps	Contagious skin disorders	Herpes Simplex
Thrombosis / Embolism	Fractures / Sprains	Other

CAUTIONS

Thrombosis/Strokes	Osteoporosis	Back/Neck problems
Aneurosa	Spondilitis	Recent operations
M.E.	Thyroid problems	Medication taken

LIFESTYLE / OTHER DETAILS

Occupation		Sleep patterns	
General Health		Allergies	
Exercise		Medication taken	
Diet		History of headaches/ migraines	
Fluid intake (water,		Emotional /	

juice)		psychological state at present	
Smoking		Stress levels	
Alcohol		Methods of relaxation	

OBJECTIVES OF THE TREATMENT & TREATMENT PLAN

What does the client hope to achieve?	
What will it be possible to achieve realistically? (Short term and long-term goals)	
Treatment plan agreed with the client (number of treatments to be given, over what period of time, length of time between treatments, areas to be paid particular attention to during the treatments)	

DISCLAIMER

I declare, that all the information regarding me in this form is true and accurate, and as far as I am aware, I can undertake a massage treatment without any adverse effects. I have been fully informed of any contra-indications and I am willing to undertake the treatment with this therapist.

Client's signature...Date..

TREATMENT DETAILS & CLIENT RESPONSE TO TREATMENT

Medium used:

Treatment 1 / Date..

Treatment 2 / Date..

Treatment 3 / Date..

Treatment 4 / Date..

Client's response / reactions to the treatments:

Treatment 1 / Date..

Treatment 2 / Date...

Treatment 3 / Date...

Treatment 4 / Date...

AFTERCARE AND GENERAL ADVICE

Treatment 1...

Treatment 2 ....

Treatment 3 ....

Treatment 4 ....

CLIENT'S FEEDBACK/ COMMENTS

Signature .... Date...

INDIAN HEAD MASSAGE CONSULTATION FORM

Therapist:	Therapist's address:	Date:
Client's name	Age	Gender
Client's address: Tel No:	Occupation:	Doctor's address/Telephone No. :

CONTRA-INDICATIONS

Diabetes	Cuts / Abrasions/recent scars	Spastic conditions
Abnormal blood pressure	Migraine	Sties
Epilepsy	Osteoporosis	Conjunctivitis
Cancer	Local infections	Advanced asthma
Undiagnosed lumps	Contagious skin disorders	Herpes Simplex
Thrombosis / Embolism	Fractures / Sprains	Other

CAUTIONS

Thrombosis/Strokes	Osteoporosis	Back/Neck problems
Aneurosa	Spondilitis	Recent operations
M.E.	Thyroid problems	Medication taken

LIFESTYLE / OTHER DETAILS

Occupation		Sleep patterns	
General Health		Allergies	
Exercise		Medication taken	
Diet		History of headaches/ migraines	
Fluid intake (water,		Emotional /	

juice)		psychological state at present	
Smoking		Stress levels	
Alcohol		Methods of relaxation	

OBJECTIVES OF THE TREATMENT & TREATMENT PLAN

What does the client hope to achieve?	
What will it be possible to achieve realistically? (Short term and long-term goals)	
Treatment plan agreed with the client (number of treatments to be given, over what period of time, length of time between treatments, areas to be paid particular attention to during the treatments)	

DISCLAIMER

I declare, that all the information regarding me in this form is true and accurate, and as far as I am aware, I can undertake a massage treatment without any adverse effects. I have been fully informed of any contra-indications and I am willing to undertake the treatment with this therapist.

Client's signature..Date...

TREATMENT DETAILS & CLIENT RESPONSE TO TREATMENT

Medium used:

Treatment 1 / Date...

Treatment 2 / Date...

Treatment 3 / Date...

Treatment 4 / Date...

Client's response / reactions to the treatments:

Treatment 1 / Date..

Treatment 2 / Date..

Treatment 3 / Date..

Treatment 4 / Date..

AFTERCARE AND GENERAL ADVICE

Treatment 1..

Treatment 2 ....

Treatment 3 ....

Treatment 4 ....

CLIENT'S FEEDBACK/ COMMENTS

Signature .... Date..

Notes

Notes

Notes

Notes

Notes

Notes

Notes

Notes

Notes

Notes

Notes

Notes

64434407R00070